The Hair Care Regimen Manual

A Step By Step Guide For Taking Care of Relaxed, Natural & Transitioning Hair

AUTHOR BREANNA RUTTER

TABLE OF CONTENTS

INTRODUCTION TO
THE HAIR CARE REGIMEN MANUAL

"The Hair Care Regimen Manual is a pocket guide that will help you by providing hair care techniques, growth advice, and hairstyles that will help you to care for your relaxed, transitioning, or natural hair. A quality hair care regimen is the key to flourishing healthy hair. Only healthy hair can truly reach longer lengths, especially if growing your hair is a major goal of yours, this manual will teach you how to grow your hair longer while at the same time, following techniques that reinforce the health of your hair.

This manual focuses on the hair care products that are needed to take care of your hair, step by step details on how to use each individual product, and ultimately a complete hair care regimen for each specific type of hair whether you are natural, transiting, or relaxed!

The skills required to implementing your hair care regimen are of a minimum skill level paired with a vast array of hair knowledge so that you can understand why you have to do certain things to your hair, to maintain and encourage the health of it. This manual is here to thoroughly educate you about your hair and what it takes to make sure that your hair is thriving through implementing a regimen.

Please enjoy this informative read and remain patient throughout the process as you are learning to care for your hair through your specific hair care regimen!"

Sincerely Breanna

1 HAIR CARE TOOLS

It should be of no surprise that the tools you use to take care of your hair whether relaxed, natural, or transitioning are extremely important in regards to maintaining healthy hair! There are a wide variety of hair care tools available on the market so don't allow yourself to become overwhelmed by their visual appeal. The most important thing to keep in mind when acquiring your hair care tools, is that they are constructed in a manner that does not compromise the health of your hair. New tools will always rise and fall and even if some actually gain popularity, there is no need to sway from your tools of choice if they meets your needs.

The only hair tool that is necessary for detangling and maintaining groomed hair, no matter the type, is a seamless wide tooth detangling comb! This has always been the #1 secret to great hair no matter how fine, thick, course, silky, curly, straight, or wavy your hair is, you will always need a wide tooth comb for your detangling & grooming needs! This tool will prevent a great deal of damage & split ends, trust me!

What's also just as important as a seamless wide tooth detangling comb, are a pair of hair cutting shears. To keep your hair in tip top condition, you have to occasionally trim damaged/splitting ends when necessary. Also since the oldest part of your hair are the ends, it's normal that overtime, you will experience splitting or slightly damaged ends even if you have very healthy hair!

I will provide a list of safe and harsh hair care tools to use on your hair whether for maintenance or styling!

SAFE HAIR CARE TOOLS	HARSH HAIR CARE TOOLS
Seamless Wide Tooth Comb	Combs with Seams In-between the Teeth
Soft Boar Bristle Hair Brush	Plastic Bristle Hair Brush
Hair Cutting Shears (only to be used on hair)	Safety Scissors (Household Scissors)
Silk Hair Accessories	Cotton/Wool Hair Accessories
Ouch less/Seamless Hair Bands	Metal Bind/Plastic Bind On Hair Bands
Paddle Brush	Metal Wig Brush
Heat Styling Up To 350°	Heat Styling Over 350°
Blow Drying on Low-Medium Heat	Blow Drying on High Heat

2 DETANGLE

Properly detangling your hair is your first line of defense when protecting yourself from breakage and damage. Use extreme gentleness when detangling your hair because the line of demarcation (refer to definition guide) with relaxed and transitioning hair is the weakest point of your hair. In regards to natural hair, rushed detangling will cause breakage no matter your curl type! When freeing tangles, you must detangle your hair with a seamless wide tooth comb at all times! Sometimes just raking your fingers gently through your hair is enough, depending on the state of your hair, but a wide tooth comb is preferred. Also, make it a priority to only detangle your hair when necessary because your chances of hair damage increases as manipulation increases. It is best to only detangle your hair prior to shampoo washing, before a hair treatment, or before styling to keep detangling at a minimum. A great way to limit your frequency of detangling is to style your hair in a way that will allow your hairstyle to last until your next co wash or shampoo wash!

Detangling your hair will differ depending on if you have relaxed, natural, or transitioning hair. Relaxed hair is best detangled on dry ends first and then your roots while wet. Transitioning hair is best detangled when done similarly to relaxed hair, and natural hair is best detangled while hair is wet with a slip agent. Straight hair should always be detangled dry, and wavy to curly hair should always be detangled wet with a slip agent.. The reason why relaxed hair should be detangled dry & your roots wet, is because relaxed hair has a tendency to tangle/mat when wet.

I will walk you step by step through how to detangle your hair properly no matter the type of hair you have!

Relaxed Hair Detangle Regimen

Step #1 Use your hands to separate relaxed hair into manageable sections for easy detangling (6 to 8 sections).

Use hair clips to help keep your hair sectioned!

Step #2 Dry detangle relaxed ends in manageable sections from the tips to the line of demarcation with a seamless wide tooth comb.

Step #3 (New Growth) Generously apply your rinse conditioner to your new growth and wait a couple of minutes until your hair has softened.

Step #4 Per section, gently detangle your new growth by starting at the line of demarcation and following through to the ends. Mist hair with water to help detangle if necessary. Continue each detangling stroke higher up your new growth until you reach your scalp. The last detangling stroke is when you can successfully comb once with ease through your section of hair!

Step #5 Loosely braid or twist each section and rinse out all traces of conditioner with warm water.

Step #6 Final rinse with the coolest water you can stand to close your cuticles for smooth frizz free hair.

Step #7 Pat towel dry, unravel your sections and proceed to follow up with styling or follow up with your hair treatment of choice!

Natural Hair Detangle Regimen

Step #1 Use your hands to separate natural hair into manageable sections for easy detangling (6 to 8 sections).

Use hair clips to help keep hair sectioned!

Step #2 Generously apply your rinse conditioner to your sections of hair and wait a couple of minutes until your hair has softened.

Step #3 Per section, start at the ends and gently detangle your hair working your way up to your scalp. Mist hair with water to help detangle if necessary.

The last detangling stroke is when you can successfully comb once with ease through your section of hair!

Step #4 Loosely braid or twist each section and rinse out all traces of conditioner with warm water.

Step #5 Final rinse with the coolest water you can stand to close your cuticles for smooth frizz free hair.

Step #6 Pat towel dry, unravel your sections and proceed to follow up with styling or follow up with your hair treatment of choice!

Transitioning Hair Detangle Regimen

Step #1 Use your hands to separate hair into manageable sections for easy detangling (6 to 8 sections).

Use hair clips to help keep hair sectioned!

Step #1 Dry detangle relaxed ends in manageable sections from the tips to the line of demarcation with a seamless wide tooth comb.

Step #3 (Natural Hair) Generously apply your rinse conditioner to your natural hair and wait a couple of minutes until your hair has softened.

Step #4 Per section, gently detangle your new growth by starting at the line of demarcation and following through to the ends. Mist hair with water to help detangle if necessary. Continue each detangling stroke higher up your natural hair until you reach your scalp. The last detangling stroke is when you can successfully comb once with ease through your section of hair!

Step #5 Loosely braid or twist each section and rinse out all traces of conditioner with warm water.

Step #6 Final rinse with the coolest water you can stand to close your cuticles for smooth frizz free hair.

Step #7 Pat towel dry, unravel your sections and proceed to follow up with styling or follow up with your hair treatment of choice!

3 SHAMPOO

When shampooing your hair, understand that a little shampoo goes a long way no matter the state of your hair! In fact, black hair does not have to be shampooed as often as other hair types and because of this, there is the added pressure of finding the perfect shampoo that will not strip your hair of vital moisture. Commercial shampoos are usually filled with very stripping cleansing agents that often leave your hair dryer than before even after shampooing!

Using a mild shampoo is all around better for preserving the health of your hair because of its mild cleansing power. Additionally, every time you shampoo wash your hair, it is highly advisable that you perform a Deep Condition Treatment but if your shampoo does not cause a squeaky clean finish, skipping a Deep Conditioning Treatment is just fine! The only type of hair that requires two different kinds of shampoo (a mild shampoo and clarifying shampoo) is relaxed hair because most relaxers contribute to mineral buildup that have to be removed. To learn in depth information about relaxers, refer to The Relaxed Hair Bible book!

Relaxed hair should be shampoo washed weekly with a mild shampoo and once a month with a clarifying shampoo while natural hair and transitioning hair should be shampooed weekly or twice a month. Shampoo washing your hair will also vary depending on how frequent you use other hair products and the condition of your scalp & hair. In any case, even if you work out, do not shampoo your hair more than once a week no matter your type of hair. Instead, conditioner wash halfway through the week until your next shampoo wash.

Shampoo wash according to your unique needs by paying attention to any buildup, odor, or itch since those are good indicators that it would be a good time to shampoo wash your hair.

I will walk you step by step through how to shampoo wash, no matter your type of hair. If you are in need of a quality shampoo, I highly suggest HowToBlackHair.com referred hair care products specifically formulated for maintaining healthy hair.

Relaxed Hair Shampoo Regimen

Step #1 Follow the Relaxed Hair Detangle Regimen but skip Steps 6 & 7.

Step #2 Apply shampoo directly to the scalp and message with finger pads to form a lather.

Step #3 Unravel a section and use lather to cleanse the ends then lightly re-braid or re-twist your section.

Repeat this step on all sections one at a time.

Step #4 Rinse all traces of shampoo from hair with warm water.

Step #5 Final rinse with the coolest water you can stand to close your cuticles for smooth frizz free hair.

Step #6 Pat towel dry, unravel your sections and proceed to follow up with styling or your treatment of choice!

Natural Hair Shampoo Regimen

Step #1 Follow the Natural Hair Detangle Regimen but skip Steps 5 & 6.

Step #2 Apply shampoo directly to the scalp and message with finger pads to form a lather.

Step #3 Unravel a section and use lather to cleanse the ends then lightly re-braid or re-twist your section.

Repeat this step on all sections one at a time.

Step #4 Rinse all traces of shampoo from hair with warm water.

Step #5 Final rinse with the coolest water you can stand to close your cuticles for smooth frizz free hair.

Step #6 Pat towel dry, unravel your sections and proceed to follow up with styling or your hair treatment of choice!

Transitioning Hair Shampoo Regimen

Step #1 Follow the Transitioning Hair Detangle Regimen but skip Steps 6 & 7.

Step #2 Apply shampoo directly to the scalp and message with finger pads to form a lather.

Step #3 Unravel a section and use lather to cleanse the ends then lightly re-braid or re-twist your section.

Repeat this step on all sections one at a time.

Step #4 Rinse all traces of shampoo from hair with warm water.

Step #5 Final rinse with the coolest water you can stand to close your cuticles for smooth frizz free hair.

Step #6 Pat towel dry, unravel your sections and proceed to follow up with styling or your hair treatment of choice!

4 DEEP CONDITION

Your hair requires deep condition treatments to keep it healthy, especially when it comes to preserving the health of hair that has a tendency to be chronically dry! Relaxed hair is the weakest of them all when it comes to dryness because the health of this hair has been compromised since relaxers strip this hair of protein and moisture. That's why a bi-monthly shaft penetrating deep conditioner is a necessary treatment you must incorporate into your regimen if you want healthy relaxed hair. Transitioning hair is also at risk of dryness and breakage since the ends are relaxed so the same frequency of deep conditioning also applies.

Using a deep condition product will not be done as frequently on natural hair but it is vital for balancing much needed moisture into your hair. You will usually notice that during the hotter & drier times of year, more deep conditioning is required for hair in any state whether relaxed, natural, or transitioning!

Relaxed hair should receive a deep condition at least twice a month as well as the relaxed portion of your transitioning hair. Natural hair should be deep conditioned at least once a month. Deep conditioning your hair can vary depending on how tight your curl pattern is, your hair care styling habits, usage of heat styling, and other hair products as well. Also, while deep conditioning your hair, remember to avoid adding product to your scalp as this can cause buildup!

Next, I will walk you step by step through how to deep condition your hair no matter the type of hair you have! If you are in need of a quality deep conditioner, I highly suggest HowToBlackHair.com referred hair care products specifically formulated for maintaining healthy hair.

Relaxed Hair Deep Condition Regimen

Step #1 Follow the Relaxed Hair Detangle Regimen but skip Steps 6 & 7.

Step #2 Generously apply your deep conditioner section by section to your hair focusing on your relaxed portion, and allow product to treat for about 30 minutes.

Re-braid or re-twist sections.

USING HEAT Cover all hair with a plastic shower cap and sit under a hooded dryer for at least 20 minutes.

Step #3 After treating for about 20 to 30 minutes, rinse out all traces of deep conditioner with warm water.

Step #4 Final rinse with the coolest water you can stand to close your cuticles for smooth frizz free hair.

Step #5 Pat towel dry, unravel your sections and proceed to follow up with styling!

Natural Hair Deep Condition Regimen

Step #1 Follow the Natural Hair Detangle Regimen but skip Steps 5 & 6.

Step #2 Generously apply your deep conditioner section by section to your hair focusing on your ends and allow product to treat for about 30 minutes.

Re-braid or re-twist sections.

USING HEAT Cover all hair with a plastic shower cap and sit under a hooded dryer for at least 20 minutes.

Step #3 After treating for about 20 to 30 minutes, rinse out all traces of deep conditioner with warm water.

Step #4 Final rinse with the coolest water you can stand to close your cuticles for smooth frizz free hair.

Step #5 Pat towel dry, unravel your sections and proceed to follow up with styling!

Transitioning Hair Deep Condition Regimen

Step #1 Follow the Transitioning Hair Detangle Regimen but skip Steps 6 & 7.

Step #2 Generously apply your deep conditioner section by section to your hair focusing on your relaxed ends and allow product to treat for about 30 minutes.

Re-braid or re-twist sections.

USING HEAT Cover all hair with a plastic shower cap and sit under a hooded dryer for at least 20 minutes.

Step #3 After treating for about 20 to 30 minutes, rinse out all traces of deep conditioner with warm water.

Step #4 Final rinse with the coolest water you can stand to close your cuticles for smooth frizz free hair.

Step #5 Pat towel dry, unravel your sections and proceed to follow up with styling!

5 PROTEIN TREATMENT

Protein treatments serve as a corrective treatment for hair that is lacking in strength. To restore elasticity on the other hand, deep conditioners specifically serve that purpose for your hair. A product formulated as a protein treatment has the ability to penetrate your hair shaft which is necessary for making hair stronger from the inside out. Relaxed and transitioning hair desperately need a protein treatment to prevent the relaxed portion of the hair from breaking! Natural hair on the other hand is stronger because it has not been stripped of its protein so using protein products aren't needed. No matter your hair, too much protein will make it stiff or crunchy to touch! Protein treatments are still to be taken with caution on relaxed and transitioning hair because hair that has too much protein will become brittle when its elasticity has been compromised.

A protein treatment (or protein deep condition treatment) needs to be performed at least twice a month and right after relaxing your hair. Along with having a protein leave in, a protein treatment should be used after rinsing your relaxer out of your hair with water which is right before washing your hair with your neutralizing shampoo. This is the perfect opportunity to treat your hair because in that moment, it is most susceptible to damage! The relaxed portion of transitioning hair should also be protein treated twice a month as well while avoiding treating the natural hair. Natural hair can be protein treated once a month but it is better to treat the hair when it feels gummy, stretchy or weak to avoid protein buildup!

I will walk you step by step through using your protein treatment! If you need a quality protein hair product, I highly suggest HowToBlackHair.com line of hair products.

Relaxed Hair Protein Treatment Regimen

Step #1 On detangled manageable sections, coat each section with your Protein Treatment/Conditioner.

(Best used RIGHT AFTER rinsing out your relaxer & RIGHT BEFORE shampooing with your neutralizing shampoo).

Step #2 Leave on hair as suggested by the product or at least for 10 minutes.

(For best penetration, sit under a hooded dryer with a plastic shower cap for 10 to 15 minutes).

Step #3 Thoroughly rinse out protein product from your hair with warm water for about 5 minutes (this is helping the PH of your hair return to its normal level).

Step #4 Proceed to shampoo your hair with your neutralizing shampoo for at least 5 minutes.

Step #5 Rinse with warm water and final rinse with the coolest water you can stand to close your cuticles for smooth frizz free hair

Step #6 Pat towel dry, unravel your sections and proceed to follow up with styling!

Natural Hair Protein Treatment Regimen

Step #1 On detangled manageable sections, coat each section with your Protein Deep Conditioner.

Step #2 Per section, saturate the ends with your protein product & loosely re-braid or re-twist each section. Protein treat as suggested by the product, or cover your hair with a shower cap to process for 30 minutes max.

*For Intense Results: cover hair with a shower cap and protein treat for a max time of 30 minutes under a hooded dryer. This is necessary in the case of treating extremely damaged hair!

Step #3 Thoroughly rinse out all traces of the protein treatment from your hair with warm water & final rinse with the coolest water you can stand to close your cuticles for smooth frizz free hair.

Step #4 Pat towel dry, unravel your sections, and proceed to follow up with your styling of choice!

Transitioning Hair Protein Treatment Regimen

Step #1 On detangled manageable sections, coat each section of relaxed hair with your Protein Deep Conditioner.

Step #2 Per section, saturate the relaxed ends with your protein treatment & loosely re-braid or re-twist each section. Protein treat as suggested by the product, or cover your hair with a shower cap to process for 30 minutes max.

*For Intense Results: cover hair with a shower cap and protein treat for a max time of 30 minutes under a hooded dryer. This is necessary in the case of treating extremely damaged hair!

Step #3 Thoroughly rinse out all traces of the protein treatment from your hair with warm water & final rinse with the coolest water you can stand to close your cuticles for smooth frizz free hair.

Step #4 Pat towel dry, unravel your sections, and proceed to follow up with your styling of choice!

6 CONDITIONER WASH

No matter if your hair is relaxed, transitioning, or natural, black hair always needs a steady supply of moisture. Healthy hair is hair that is kept moisturized, as this prevents it from becoming dry which leads to splitting breaking ends! The key to any successful hair care regimen believe it or not is an incorporation of co washing. Co wash means to wash your hair with conditioner alone and this is a great way to moisturize your hair when you are noticing that your hair is becoming dry but is not quite ready for a shampoo wash.

Its preferred to use an inexpensive water based conditioning product to serve as your co wash conditioner as well as to aid you with detangling. Rinse Conditioners/Co Wash Conditioners are usually used frequently and in large quantities so having an adequate supply of this conditioner is important when helping you maintain the health of your hair.

Co wash natural, relaxed, and transitioning hair at least weekly or occasionally twice a week if needed. Depending on the moisture needs of your hair, especially in regards to natural hair, co washing twice a week is also acceptable. Those who are physically active whether it be sports or working out, co washing your hair twice a week is helpful when managing the health of your hair and scalp to avoid a buildup of dirt and sweat.

I will walk you step by step through how to co-wash your hair and if you are in need of a quality conditioner, I highly suggest HowToBlackHair.com referred hair care products specifically formulated for maintaining healthy hair.

Relaxed Hair Conditioner Wash Regimen

Step #1 Dry detangle relaxed ends in manageable sections (6-8 sections) from the tips to your scalp with a seamless wide tooth comb.

Step #2 Loosely braid or twist each section after detangling.

Step #3 Saturate your hair with warm water and generously apply your rinse conditioner to each section of your hair focusing on your relaxed ends.

Step #4 Re-braid and re-twist sections after applying conditioner.

Step #5 Rinse conditioner from hair with warm water.

Step #6 Final rinse with the coolest water you can stand to close your cuticles for smooth frizz free hair.

Step #7 Pat towel dry, unravel your sections and proceed to follow up with styling!

Natural Hair Conditioner Wash Regimen

Step #1 Saturate your hair with warm water and generously apply your rinse conditioner to each section of your hair focusing on your ends.

Step #2 Loosely braid or twist sections after applying conditioner.

Step #3 Use a seamless wide tooth detangling comb to detangle each section.

Step #4 Continue each detangling stroke higher up until you reach your scalp. The last detangling stroke is when you can successfully comb once with ease through your section of hair!

Step #5 Rinse conditioner from hair with warm water.

Step #6 Final rinse with the coolest water you can stand to close your cuticles for smooth frizz free hair.

Step #7 Pat towel dry, unravel your sections and proceed to follow up with styling!

Transitioning Hair Conditioner Wash Regimen

Step #1 Dry detangle relaxed ends in manageable sections (6-8 sections) from the tips to your line of demarcation with a seamless wide tooth comb.

Step #2 Saturate your hair with warm water and generously apply your rinse conditioner to each section of your hair focusing on your ends.

Step #3 Loosely braid or twist sections after applying conditioner.

Step #4 Use a seamless wide tooth detangling comb to detangle each section.

Continue each detangling stroke higher up until you reach your scalp.

The last detangling stroke is when you can successfully comb once with ease through your section of hair!

Step #5 Rinse conditioner from hair with warm water.

Step #6 Final rinse with the coolest water you can stand to close your cuticles for smooth frizz free hair.

Step #7 Pat towel dry, unravel your sections and proceed to follow up with styling!

7 LEAVE IN MOISTURIZER

A leave in moisturizer (conditioner) is a mandatory hair care product you will need to assist your hair care regimen because keeping your hair moisturized allows you to maintain healthy hair. The absence of your leave in moisturizer will leave your hair constantly on the edge of dryness and prone to breakage and splitting ends. Also, it is very important that your moisturizer does not contain proteins because you are already receiving adequate protein from your protein treatment/conditioner.

A leave in moisturizer needs to be used at least twice a week with transitioning, natural, and relaxed hair. Some of the best times to use this moisturizer is right after shampooing and before styling your hair. If you do not moisturize your hair before styling, you can cause breakage that could have been easily prevented had you moisturized!

With this product, you have to experiment applying it on damp or dry hair to find out when applying it to your hair is best. Many with transitioning or natural hair prefer applying a leave in on damp hair because it feels like the product actually absorbs into the hair rather than sit on top of their strands. If you have problems with dry hair, try applying your leave in moisturizer with the LOC method. Refer to the definition guide for more information on the LOC Method!

I will walk you step by step through how to moisturize your hair and if you are in need of a quality leave in moisturizer, I highly suggest HowToBlackHair.com referred hair care products specifically formulated for maintaining healthy hair.

Relaxed Hair Leave In Moisturizer Regimen

Step #1 Follow the Relaxed Hair Detangle Regimen but allow hair to air dry fully or partially while in sections.

Step #2 Coat leave in moisturizer, section by section, on detangled hair.

Do not apply product to the scalp as this can cause buildup!

Step #3 For increased moisture (if you struggle with dry hair) incorporate the LOC Method with your choice of hair care products.

Step #4 Proceed to style working on one section at a time.

If you like to style dried hair, allow hair to air dry or blow dry preferably with low heat.

Natural Hair Leave In Moisturizer Regimen

Step #1 Follow the Natural Hair Detangle Regimen but allow hair to air dry fully or partially while in sections.

Step #2 Coat leave in moisturizer, section by section, on detangled hair.

Do not apply product to the scalp as this can cause buildup!

Step #3 For increased moisture (if you struggle with dry hair) incorporate the LOC Method with your choice of hair care products.

Step #4 Proceed to style working on one section at a time.

If you like to style dried hair, allow hair to air dry or blow dry preferably with low heat.

Transitioning Hair Leave In Moisturizer Regimen

Step #1 Follow the Transitioning Hair Detangle Regimen but allow hair to air dry fully or partially while in sections.

Step #2 Coat leave in moisturizer, section by section, on detangled hair.

Do not apply product to the scalp as this can cause buildup!

Step #3 For increased moisture (if you struggle with dry hair) incorporate the LOC Method with your choice of hair care products.

Step #4 Proceed to style working on one section at a time.

If you like to style dried hair, allow hair to air dry or blow dry preferably with low heat.

8 OIL SEALANT

Your choice of an oil sealant will prevent your moisturizing practices from being a waste of time and effort! Throughout this manual, there has been an extreme emphasis placed on keeping your hair supplied with moisture because healthy hair is synonymous with moisturized hair. The purpose of using an oil sealant in your hair care regimen, is to slow down the rate of water evaporating from the strands of your hair. To clarify, there is no such thing as a permanent sealant that will keep your hair moisturized forever because a sealant like that will most likely damage your hair, prevent you from effectively using heat, and make chemical treatments like coloring and deep conditioning ineffective. Keep in mind that the heavier or thicker your oil sealant of choice is, the longer your hair can retain moisture and the more greasy your hair may feel.

Use an oil sealant on your hair, whether natural, relaxed, or transitioning before or after applying your leave in moisturizer. If you adopt the LOC Method, sealing your hair with oil will be done before your creamy leave in moisturizer is applied to your hair. Depending on your hair, you may prefer lighter oils like Coconut oil or heavier oils/butters like Castor oil or Shea Butter. For the majority, tighter curl patterns lean more towards heavier oils/butters and looser curl patterns, lean more towards lighter oils. If your hair has a tendency to have a constant dryness, try thicker consistency (heavier) oils/butters and if you don't have much difficulty maintaining moisturized hair, try thinner consistency (lighter) oils as your oil sealant.

I will walk you step by step through how to oil seal your hair and if you are in need of a quality oil sealant, I highly suggest HowToBlackHair.com referred hair care products specifically formulated for maintaining healthy hair.

Relaxed, Natural, and Transitioning
Hair Oil Sealant Regimen

Step #1 (Without the LOC Method)

Lightly coat fingers with your oil/butter of choice and lubricate damp hair in manageable sections at a time.

Oil seal preferably AFTER applying your creamy leave in moisturizer or oil seal on damp product free hair.

Focus on the ends of your hair as this needs the most coverage when maintaining moisturized hair!

Step #2 (With the LOC Method)

Lightly coat fingers with your oil/butter of choice and lubricate manageable sections at a time RIGHT BEFORE applying your creamy leave in moisturizer.

After applying your oil, apply your creamy leave in moisturizer to complete the LOC Method.

Step #3 Proceed to style working on one section at a time.

If you like to style dried hair, allow hair to air dry or blow dry preferably with low heat.

9 HAIR GEL

Hair gel is an optional hair product unlike your other hair care products. The previous hair products mentioned are mandatory for a healthy hair care regimen but products like gel, mousse, or holding sprays are 100% optional when you want to use them for styling. Your choice of hair gel in particular, will depend on your styling needs and how well your hair gel will cooperate with your hair products. For a light hold, watery/loose consistency hair gels can provide a little hold but for keeping edges held smooth and slick without waving or reverting to curls, a stronger hold (thicker consistency) gel would be better. Gels can be used to keep your hair slick and smooth and this product can also be used to define your hair to make your curl pattern pop!

How often you should use hair gel depends on your styling needs. The consistency and hold of your hair gel are not synonymous with being best for certain hair textures or curl patterns. Some gels provide light, medium, or strong holds according to their labels. Only apply hair gel to moisturized hair to avoid hard hair and be cautious of gels that contain protein in their ingredients list. Using hair gel with protein as an ingredient is an easy way to overload your hair so to avoid this, avoid proteins in your gel.

I will walk you step by step through how to use hair gel on your hair and if you are in need of a quality hair gel, I highly suggest HowToBlackHair.com referred hair care products specifically formulated for maintaining healthy hair.

Relaxed, Natural, and Transitioning Hair Gel Regimen

Step #1 Lightly coat fingers with your hair gel and lubricate manageable sections at a time then proceed to style!

This step is great for curl sets like; Perm Rod Sets, Straw Sets, or Flexi rod Sets for example!

SCULPTED EDGES Apply your hair gel to your edges and sculpt with the pads of your fingers or a soft toothbrush (commonly used).

OPTIONAL Tie down your hair (or edges) with a silk head scarf or a molding strip for at least 5 minutes.

This allows your hair to set while drying.

10 HAIR CARE REGIMEN

I have explained the purpose of your hair care products, how often to apply them and more importantly, directions on how to apply them! Each hair care regimen will slightly differ depending on the health of each unique type of hair. With patience and a little skill, you will be able to take great care of your hair no matter if you decide to have natural hair, relaxed hair or transition hair. As you may have observed, taking care of your hair has to always be done in sections being that there is a preferred way to prevent excessive combing while detangling. Understanding how to do a variety of simple hair care techniques all contribute to your overall hair care regimen.

So of course it's almost a given that you still don't understand how to implement an overall regimen that will work for your specific type of hair. Each suggested product regimen can make you feel overwhelmed about how to handle and care for your hair!

Follow along with the suggested weekly hair care regimen that will be explained next and keep in mind that the chart is 100% flexible to your unique hair care needs. One day you may feel the need to tweak certain parts of the hair care regimen so feel free to make changes that are necessary for you.

I will walk you step by step through an awesome hair care regimen that you can use as a guide for taking care of your transitioning, relaxed, or natural hair and in the following sections, we will discuss the topic on using relaxers, hairstyling options, and so much more!

THE RELAXED HAIR CARE REGIMEN
(FRESHLY RELAXED HAIR)

(WEEK 1 / DAY 1)	(WEEK 2 / DAY 1)
*Shampoo *Protein Treatment (Conditioner) *Leave In Moisturizer *Hair Gel (optional)	*Shampoo *Deep Condition *Protein Leave In *Hair Gel (optional)
(WEEK 1 / DAY 2)	(WEEK 2 / DAY 2)
(WEEK 1 / DAY 3)	(WEEK 2 / DAY 3)
(WEEK 1 / DAY 4) *Protein Leave In	(WEEK 2 / DAY 4) *Leave In Moisturizer
(WEEK 1 / DAY 5)	(WEEK 2 / DAY 5)
(WEEK 1 / DAY 6) *Leave In Moisturizer	(WEEK 2 / DAY 6) *Protein Leave In
(WEEK 1 / DAY 7)	(WEEK 2 / DAY 7)

Deep Condition Twice A Month
Protein Treat Twice A Month (If Necessary)

Feel free to moisturize more frequently if necessary.

NATURAL HAIR CARE REGIMEN

(WEEK 1 / DAY 1)	(WEEK 2 / DAY 1)
*Shampoo *Leave In Moisturizer *Oil Sealant *Hair Gel (optional)	*Leave In Moisturizer *Oil Sealant *Hair Gel (optional)
(WEEK 1 / DAY 2)	(WEEK 2 / DAY 2)
(WEEK 1 / DAY 3)	(WEEK 2 / DAY 3)
(WEEK 1 / DAY 4) *Co wash *Leave In Moisturizer *Oil Sealant *Hair Gel (optional)	(WEEK 2 / DAY 4) *Co wash *Leave In Moisturizer *Oil Sealant *Hair Gel (optional)
(WEEK 1 / DAY 5)	(WEEK 2 / DAY 5)
(WEEK 1 / DAY 6)	(WEEK 2 / DAY 6)
(WEEK 1 / DAY 7) *Leave In Moisturizer	(WEEK 1 / DAY 7) *Leave In Moisturizer

Deep Condition Once A Month
Protein Treat Once A Month (If Necessary)

Feel free to moisturize more frequently if necessary

TRANSITIONING HAIR CARE REGIMEN

(WEEK 1/DAY 1)	(WEEK 2/DAY 1)
*Shampoo *Protein Treatment (Conditioner) *Leave In Moisturizer *Hair Gel (optional)	*Shampoo *Deep Condition *Protein Leave In *Hair Gel (optional)
(WEEK 1/DAY 2)	(WEEK 2/DAY 2)
(WEEK 1/DAY 3)	(WEEK 2/DAY 3)
(WEEK 1/DAY 4) *Co Wash *Leave In Moisturizer *Oil Sealant *Hair Gel (optional)	(WEEK 2/DAY 4) *Co Wash *Leave In Moisturizer *Oil Sealant *Hair Gel (optional)
(WEEK 1/DAY 5)	(WEEK 2/DAY 5)
(WEEK 1/DAY 6)	(WEEK 2/DAY 6)
(WEEK 1/DAY 7) *Leave In Moisturizer	(WEEK 1/DAY 7) *Leave In Moisturizer

Deep Condition Twice A Month
Protein Treat Relaxed Ends Twice A Month (If Necessary)

Feel free to moisturize more frequently if necessary

11 CHEMICAL RELAXER

Some of those who are reading this manual may have relaxed hair and it's important to understand the effects chemical relaxers have on the health of your hair whether you have been informed or not. Always use chemical relaxers with caution and stretch your touch ups as far apart from one another as possible because breakage and thinning is always a risk when chemically relaxing your hair!

Chemical relaxers as well as their benefits and downfalls are heavily discussed in my book, The Relaxed Hair Bible: The 10 Commandments of Long Healthy Relaxed Hair so if you want to learn concentrated information on their usage, regimens, hair care treatments and more, refer to that book for detailed information. It's very important to understand the dangers of using chemical relaxers while creating a hair care regimen because the nature of relaxed hair is different than your hair in its natural chemical free state.

As discussed in the Relaxed Hair Bible, chemical relaxers are highly alkaline and by nature, they disintegrate (or break down) your hairs to the point of straightness. When a relaxer is left on for too long or too high of strength is used, this can cause your hair to melt or simply break off or begin to thin. As mentioned in previous hair care manuals, hair is best healthy when kept in the PH range of 4.5 to 5.5 and relaxers have a PH range of 11-14! This is highly corrosive but is used to caused permanent "controlled damage" to your hair and because of this, taking care of your hair in its relaxed state requires detailed precise care on your part to make sure that your hair remains healthy!

12 HAIRSTYLING OPTIONS

There are a multitude of hairstyling options you can wear with your relaxed, transitioning, and natural hair whether or not you chose to wear hair extensions. Before we get into the different kinds of hairstyles you can wear with your hair, lets first talk about how hairstyles contribute to the health of your hair and the pros and cons of various kinds of styles.

Hairstyles are a great way to encourage length retention because it limits the amount of times you have to manipulate and detangle your hair throughout the week. If you like to wear styles with or without added hair, hairstyling is a great way to look stylish while also protecting your hair from constant or daily manipulation. For many who want to grow their hair to longer lengths, protective styling protects your hair from constant heat or strain.

Protective Style: a heat free hairstyle that can be worn with or without extensions with the focus of concealing the ends of your hair with styles like buns for example which tucks and conceals your ends

The pros to wearing hairstyles of course provides length retention and low maintenance as benefits towards maintaining healthy hair. Hairstyles that require heat from tools like a straighter or blow dryer for example, dries your hair out and dry hair is the entryway to breakage so these tools should always be taken with caution!

WEAVES AND EXTENSIONS

Weaves and extensions come in different varieties such as Cold Fusions, Hot Fusions, but most popularly, Weft Extensions. When you hear someone describe their hair as a weave, it is safe to assume that the person is wearing weft extensions and there are many ways to wear these extensions with styles like; U Part Wig, Invisible Part Sew In, or a Net Weave Full Sew In for example.

Braids come in different varieties such as Yarn Braids, Cornrows, and Zillions for example. Braids can be fashioned to leave the scalp (individuals) or form against your scalp (Dutch or French braids). Some braided hairstyles that would look amazing with any type of hair like; Cornrow Extensions, Single Braids or Jumbo Braids for example.

Twists come in different varieties whether or not you chose to wear extensions with your twists or not. Twists can be fashioned against your scalp like Flat Twists or twists can leave your scalp like Two Strand Twists. Some suggested twist hairstyles that you can wear if you want to incorporate extensions are styles like; Kinky Twist, Senegalese Twist, or Havana Twist for example.

There are so many different kinds of ways you can wear your hair. Some of these hairstyles that were suggested require extensions to achieve the look and if you have long relaxed hair, some of these styles can be achieved without hair extensions instead.

DEEP WAVES

(No Heat) Take chunky sections of damp moisturized hair & secure wave rollers onto your sections. You can also achieve waves by braiding chunky braids on damp moisturized hair & unravel them when dry.

PERM ROD SET

(No Heat) Take sections of damp moisturized hair a little less wide than your perm rod & rotate the perm rod on your ends first (using gel is optional for curls with hold). After rolling the end of your section in a way that tucks your ends, continue rolling hair against the surface of the rod. Secure the plunger & allow hair to dry overnight as you sleep in a silk scarf or bonnet. Unravel rods in the opposite direction as to not disturb your curls. If desired, separate each curl for bigger hair!

FLEXI ROD SET

(No Heat) Take small to medium sections of damp moisturized hair & rotate the flexi on your ends. After rolling the end of your section in a way that tucks your ends, continue rolling hair against the surface of the flexi. Fold the top of the flexi downward, over your hair, to secure & allow hair to dry overnight. Unravel flexi rods in the opposite direction as to not disturb your curls. If desired, separate each curl for bigger hair!

For more hairstyling options, visit our hair care & styling website at HowToBlackHair.com!

13 HEAT DAMAGE

The fastest way to heat damage your hair and cause massive breakage is by using heat frequently or inappropriately! Heat damaged hair is common with many who use heat frequently, especially those who transition from relaxed hair to natural hair. Using heat to blend the two different textures of transitioning hair is a double edge sword that gives you consistent texture but on the other hand, leaves you prone to heat damage and breakage!

Heat damaged hair is easily noticed on hair that has some type of wave or curl pattern because you will notice your pattern has loosened or your pattern has not returned at all. Naturally straight or relaxed hair on the other hand feels dry or lacks in strength since heat damaged hair usually feels gummy or stretchy. Protein treatments/conditioners and deep conditioning treatments reconstruct heat damaged hair back to healthy hair in some cases. Perform a deep conditioning treatment to heat damaged hair and if you notice improvements in the health of your hair, continue deep conditioning treatments until your hair becomes healthy again. Protein treatments are the last resort to restoring hair to avoid a buildup of protein. If hair does not restored to its expected state of health, a trim is required!

Heat styling can change the structure of your hair causing it to become permanently straightened. Some individuals can tolerate a heat temperature of 350°and another individual cannot go over 300° not because their hair is unhealthy, but because everyone's hair has a different level of heat tolerance. It is not suggested to use heat on transitioning hair, even at safe temperatures, because your relaxed and natural hair has a different level of tolerance.

If you must use heat, seldom is best but all in all, styling your hair without heat will work best for you in the long run towards healthy hair.

I will walk you step by step through using heat safely on your hair, if you must. If you are in need of a quality heat protectant, I highly suggest HowToBlackHair.com referred hair care products specifically formulated for maintaining healthy hair.

Relaxed, Transitioning and Natural
Heat Protectant Regimen

THIS IS ONLY SAFE ON HEALTHY HAIR THAT IS NOT CHONICALLY DRY OR EXPERIENCING BREAKAGE!

Step #1 Prepare hair with a Protein Treatment/Condition to protect your hair.

(For best penetration, sit under a hooded dryer with a plastic shower cap for 10 to 15 minutes)

Step #2 After a thorough rinse, apply a VERY LIGHT application of Leave In Moisturizer in manageable sections.

Step #3 Once hair is dry, in manageable sections, apply a generous amount of your Heat Protectant onto your hair.

Step #4 Proceed with styling your hair with your choice of heat styling tools.

(For best healthy hair practices, use only one necessary heat source so instead of blow drying your hair, air dry and then use a straightener OR a heat curling tool to achieve your desired look).

14 TRIMMING ENDS

Trimming your ends is not to be feared because it reinforces your efforts of length retention!

Length Retention: using a collection of hair care practices and habits to grow your hair constantly towards longer lengths

Some people think that cutting your ends slows down your rate of hair growth when in all actuality, it encourages you to have more length of hair overtime.

Picture this for example, would you rather have back length stringy hair or shoulder length full hair? If you chose back length stringy hair, you are in trouble because you won't have back length hair for long! Stringy hair is the visual result of untrimmed ends and untrimmed ends will continue to break because those ends are splitting and are damaged. Long hair can be retained and actually achieved if you keep damaged splitting ends trimmed. Opt for shoulder length full hair instead because you will achieve back length full hair in time. Hair grows an average rate of 1/2 an inch a month so if you have shoulder length hair (about 12 inches) you can have back length hair (about 18 inch hair) in about a year on average. In some cases, you may grow hair at a faster rate than the average rate of growth because of variables like genetics, healthy food choices, and great hair care practices, which can contribute to longer hair in a shorter amount of time.

Trimming transitioning hair is also very important as this brings you one step closer to 100% natural hair. Transitioning hair has to eventually come to an end and it doesn't have to be done drastically, but ridding of your relaxed ends should be an important goal to achieve with your own level of comfort.

Even though your seamless wide tooth detangling comb is your most important hair tool, your cutting shears are just as important because it provides healthy ends as well as take you one step closer to your natural hair if you are transitioning!

As mentioned previously, trimming your ends does not mean that you have to big chop whatsoever, you just have to gradually trim your ends to your level of comfort. Some transitioners like to trim their hair in line of maintaining their length. For example, say you have been transitioning and you have grown 5 inches of new growth (stretched) with 10 inches of relaxed hair. Some will trim off 5 inches of relaxed hair if they have reached 5 inches of new growth, which leaves you with 10 inches of 100% natural hair.

The surprise that comes along with doing this is that your hair will look significantly shorter with 10 inches of natural hair in comparison to 10 inches of relaxed hair because of shrinkage! Natural hair can shrink in length anywhere from 30% to 70% of your actual length of hair so 10 inches of un-stretched natural hair will look like 3 to 7 inches of hair! For an easier adjustment, trim off about a 1/4 inch of relaxed hair per 1 inch of new growth gain.

I will walk you step by step through how to trim your ends as well as trim damaged hair!

Relaxed, Transitioning, and Natural Hair Trimming

ONLY USE CUTTING SHEARS EXCLUSIVELY ON YOUR TRANSITIONING HAIR!

(TRIMMING RELAXED & NATURAL ENDS)

Step #1 Dust trim detangled ends while damp in small sections at a time, making sure to do so in a well lit room with mirrors to help.

Step #2 Starting in the back of your head, part a horizontal line of hair at the nape of your neck and use gator clips or duck bill clips to keep the rest of your hair sectioned out of the way. Always dust trim small sections at a time.

Step #3 Take a small section of detangled hair, twist to the ends, and trim about an 1/8 inch of hair to dust for maintenance. Your dusted hair ends should look like little flecks of hair. For a trim that requires more than an 1/8 of length lost, consult with a professional to aid you so that you don't accidently give yourself an uneven trim.

(TRIMMING TRANSITIONING HAIR)

Step #1 First decide how much length of relaxed hair you are willing to lose because losing a lot of relaxed hair at once can be difficult to deal with.

Step #2 Follow Step 2 from above but trim off your desired length. If you feel as though you need assistance, consult with a professional to aid you so that you don't accidently give yourself an uneven trim or haircut!

AFTERWORDS

"This manual was created for individuals who desire healthier hair and need detailed information on how to create a hair care regimen dedicated to their specific type of hair. Relaxed hair, transitioning hair, and natural hair all require an adequate supply of moisture (water) with an occasional supply of protein to keep the hair healthy. This is why it was fitting to explain each similar hair care regimen in one hair care manual!

Knowing how to take care of your hair, no matter what state it's in, is the key to every successful hair care journey because the key elements to healthy flourishing hair involves the incorporation of basic hair care practices. Gentle detangling, deep conditioning, co washing, shampooing, moisturizing, and trimming are the ultimate basics, and tweaking their frequencies to your unique hair care needs is perfect for your personal hair goals. Some individuals want healthier hair, some want longer hair, and truthfully some wish to have hair. Whether many realize or not, it is a blessing to have the adornment of hair on your head that many wish to have, while others easily take it for granted.

As you may have read throughout these chapters, this manual is condensed with priceless information for helping you successfully develop your hair care regimen. This collection of information will give you ultimate success with caring for your hair in the best way possible! For detailed information specifically focused on your type of hair, check out the following books; The Natural Hair Bible, The Relaxed Hair Bible, and The Transitioning Hair Manual. I hope that you thoroughly enjoyed this read, it was a pleasure of mine to write this for your knowledge and enjoyment!" Sincerely, Breanna

ADDITIONAL RESOURCES

The Official Website: www.Howtoblackhair.com

The Online Store: www.HowtoblackhairStore.com

Free Subscription Email: http://eepurl.com/FZs5b

For Additional Hair Questions

YourHairQuestions@Gmail.com

Black Hair Styling Tutorials

BlackWomenHair YouTube Channel

www.Youtube.com/BlackWomenHair

HowToBlackHair YouTube Channel

www.Youtube.com/HowToBlackHair

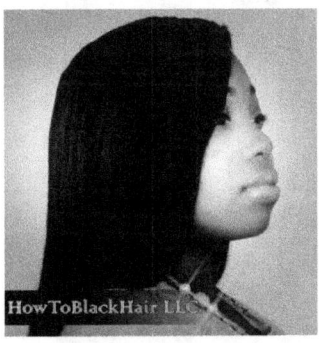

The Natural Hair Bible

The 10 Commandments of Black Hair Care

www.HowToBlackHair.com

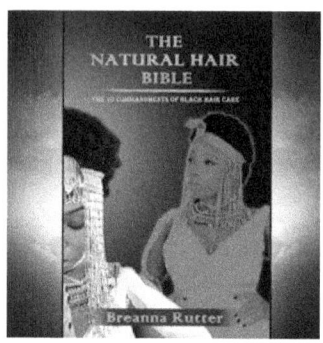

The Relaxed Hair Bible

The 10 Commandments of Long Healthy Relaxed Hair

www.HowToBlackHair.com

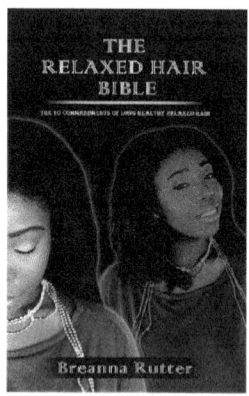

Black Hair Styling DVDs (Over 20+ Hairstyles)

www.HowToBlackHair.com

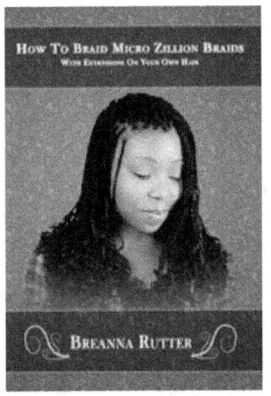 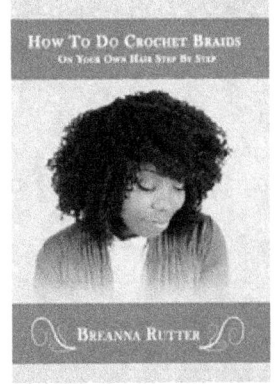

DEFINITION GUIDE

Big Chop: *drastically cutting off relaxed hair without allowing yourself to transition with occasional trims towards natural hair*

Co Wash: *washing your hair with conditioner alone*

Curl Type: *the natural curl pattern of your hair strands according to the LOIS or Andre Walker hair typing system*

Cuticles: *a naturally protecting shield (arranged like shingles to the roof of a home) outside of your hair strands*

Elasticity: *the stretching ability of your hair*

Fine Hair: *your individual strands of hair are closer in size (circumference) to string instead of thread*

Heat Tolerance: *the amount of heat handled by your hair ranging from 300° to 350°*

Lather: *using water to produce a foam with your hair care products*

Length Retention: *using a collection of hair care practices and habits to grow your hair constantly towards longer lengths*

Line Of Demarcation: *the meeting point of division between relaxed hair and natural hair or color treated hair and natural hair color*

LOC Method: *layering products for moisture in the order of; Liquid (leave in moisturizer or water), Oil, Cream (thick consistency moisturizer/sealant like a hair butter).*

Mineral Buildup: *a buildup of minerals on your hair shaft that causes rough or dry hair*

Neutralizing Shampoo: *an acidic shampoo that brings hair closer or to its natural PH (4.5 to 5.5)*

New Growth: *distinguishable unrelaxed hair growth whether relaxed or natural*

PH Range: *the alkalinity or acidity a solution is ranging from a number spectrum, of 1 (acidic) and 14 (alkaline) with water (7) being neutral*

Protective Style: *a heat free hairstyle that can be worn with or without extensions with the focus of concealing the ends of your hair with styles like buns for example*

Slip Agent: *a hair care product filled with conditioners or oils that make your hair feel slippery*

Touch Up: *relaxer treating your new growth of at least 1/4 to 1/2 an inch of unrelaxed hair*

Shrinkage: *curly hair that draws in towards a shorter length when in contact with moisture (water)*

INDEX

HOW TO BLACK HAIR LLC.
WRITTEN BY BREANNA RUTTER
BOOK DESIGNED BY BREANNA RUTTER
COVER DESIGNED BY JARED RUTTER
ALL RIGHTS RESERVED.
VISIT WWW.HOWTOBLACKHAIR.COM

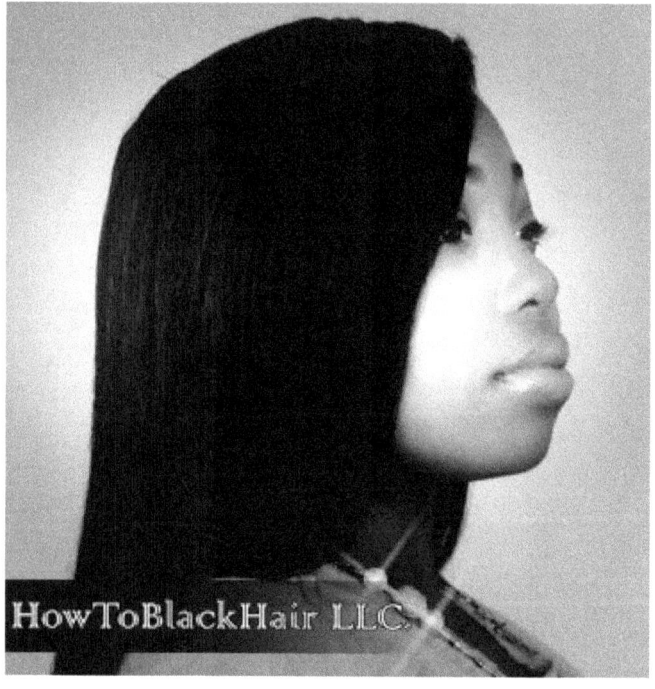